Diabetes Essential Nutrients:

10 Diabetes Friendly Snacks to Keep Blood Sugar Stable Between Meals, With a 30 Minutes Recipes Plan. Includes Cooking Tips For Beginners

Maria Spooner

Table of content

Introduction

Chapter 1: Understanding Diabetes and Blood Sugar Management

Chapter 2: The Importance of Essential Nutrients for Stable Blood Sugar

Chapter 3: Feature

Chapter 4: Why These Snacks Work for Blood Sugar Stability

Chapter 5: Benefits of Incorporating These Snacks into Your Diet

Conclusion: Empowerment Through Nutritious Snacking

Introduction

In today's fast-paced world, maintaining stable blood sugar levels can feel like an ongoing battle. Whether you're managing diabetes or simply striving for optimal health, the importance of balanced blood sugar cannot be overstated. It serves as a cornerstone for overall well-being, influencing everything from energy levels to mood stability and long-term health outcomes.

Welcome to "Essential Nutrients: 10 Diabetes-Friendly Snacks to Keep Blood Sugar Stable Between Meals." This book is not just a collection of recipes; it's a comprehensive guide designed to empower you on your journey towards better blood sugar management and overall health.

So, are you ready to take the first step towards better blood sugar management and overall health? Join me on this journey as we explore the power of essential nutrients and delicious, diabetes-friendly snacks. Let's embark on this path together and empower ourselves to thrive, one snack at a time.

Chapter 1: Understanding Diabetes and Blood Sugar Management

Diabetes is a chronic condition characterised by elevated blood sugar levels resulting from either the body's inability to produce insulin (Type 1 diabetes) or the body's ineffective use of insulin (Type 2 diabetes). It is a widespread health concern affecting millions of individuals worldwide and requires careful management to prevent complications and maintain overall health.

The Basics of Diabetes

Diabetes occurs when the body's blood sugar levels, also known as blood glucose, are consistently elevated. Glucose is a type of sugar that serves as the primary source of energy for cells throughout the body. Insulin, a hormone produced by the pancreas, plays a crucial role in regulating blood sugar levels by facilitating the uptake of glucose into cells.

In Type 1 diabetes, the immune system mistakenly attacks and destroys the insulin-producing cells in the pancreas, leading to a complete deficiency of insulin. As a result, individuals with Type 1 diabetes require lifelong insulin therapy to survive.

On the other hand, Type 2 diabetes is characterised by insulin resistance, where the body's cells become less responsive to insulin's effects. This causes blood sugar levels to rise, leading to a variety of health complications if left unmanaged. Type 2 diabetes is often associated with lifestyle factors such as obesity, poor diet, and lack of physical activity.

Blood Sugar Regulation

Maintaining stable blood sugar levels is essential for overall health and well-being. When blood sugar levels are too high (hyperglycemia) or too low (hypoglycemia), it can lead to a range of symptoms and complications.

The body employs a complex system of checks and balances to regulate blood sugar levels. After consuming a meal, the digestive system breaks down carbohydrates into glucose, which enters the bloodstream. In response, the pancreas releases insulin to facilitate the uptake of glucose into cells, where it is used for energy or stored for future use.

Conversely, when blood sugar levels drop, the pancreas releases another hormone called glucagon, which signals the liver to release stored glucose into the bloodstream to maintain optimal levels. This delicate balance ensures that cells receive a steady supply of energy while preventing blood sugar levels from spiking or crashing.

Risk Factors and Complications

Several factors can increase the risk of developing diabetes, including genetics, age, obesity, physical inactivity, and poor dietary habits. Additionally, certain medical conditions and medications may also predispose individuals to diabetes.

Uncontrolled diabetes can lead to a range of complications affecting various organs and systems in the body. Chronic hyperglycemia can damage blood vessels and nerves, leading to cardiovascular disease, kidney damage, vision loss, and nerve damage (neuropathy). Furthermore, poorly managed diabetes increases the risk of developing infections and delays wound healing.

Diagnosis and Monitoring

Diabetes is diagnosed through blood tests that measure fasting blood glucose levels, oral glucose tolerance, or glycated haemoglobin (HbA1c) levels. Regular monitoring of blood sugar levels is essential for managing diabetes effectively and preventing complications.

Individuals with diabetes may use blood glucose metres to monitor their blood sugar levels at home. These devices provide real-time feedback on blood sugar levels, allowing individuals to adjust their diet, medication, and lifestyle as needed to maintain optimal blood sugar control.

Treatment Options

Treatment for diabetes typically involves a combination of lifestyle modifications, medication, and insulin therapy. Lifestyle modifications such as adopting a healthy diet, engaging in regular physical activity, maintaining a healthy weight, and quitting smoking can help improve blood sugar control and reduce the risk of complications.

Medications such as oral antidiabetic drugs and injectable insulin may be prescribed to lower blood sugar levels and improve insulin sensitivity. Additionally, some individuals with Type 1 diabetes may require continuous subcutaneous insulin infusion (insulin pump therapy) to deliver insulin throughout the day.

Chapter 2: The Importance of Essential Nutrients for Stable Blood Sugar

Maintaining stable blood sugar levels is essential for overall health and well-being, especially for individuals managing diabetes. While medication and lifestyle factors play a significant role in blood sugar management, the role of essential nutrients should not be overlooked. In this chapter, we will explore the importance of essential nutrients in supporting stable blood sugar levels and their impact on overall health.

Understanding Essential Nutrients

Essential nutrients are compounds that the body cannot produce on its own and must be obtained through diet. These nutrients play crucial roles in various physiological processes, including energy metabolism, cellular function, and overall health. Essential nutrients include carbohydrates, proteins, fats, vitamins, minerals, and water.

Carbohydrates and Blood Sugar

Carbohydrates are the body's primary source of energy and have the most significant impact on blood sugar levels. When consumed, carbohydrates are broken down into glucose, which enters the bloodstream and raises blood sugar levels. However, not all carbohydrates are created equal.

Simple carbohydrates, such as sugar and refined grains, are quickly digested and absorbed, leading to rapid spikes in blood sugar levels. On the other hand, complex carbohydrates, found in whole grains, fruits, vegetables, and legumes, are digested more slowly, resulting in a gradual increase in blood sugar levels.

Fibre

Fibre is a type of carbohydrate that the body cannot digest, but it plays a crucial role in blood sugar management. Soluble fibre, found in foods like oats, beans, and fruits, forms a gel-like substance in the digestive tract, which slows down the absorption of glucose into the bloodstream. This helps prevent spikes in blood sugar levels and promotes overall blood sugar stability.

Additionally, fibre helps promote safety and supports digestive health, making it an essential nutrient for individuals managing diabetes.

Protein

Protein is another essential nutrient that plays a vital role in blood sugar management. When consumed, protein is broken down into amino acids, which are used by the body for various functions, including building and repairing tissues.

Unlike carbohydrates, protein has minimal impact on blood sugar levels when consumed. However, including protein-rich foods in meals and snacks can help promote safety and prevent rapid fluctuations in blood sugar levels.

Fats

While fats are often demonised in the context of blood sugar management, they play a crucial role in overall health and should be included as part of a balanced diet. Healthy fats, such as those found in avocados, nuts, seeds, and olive oil, can help improve insulin sensitivity and promote blood sugar stability when consumed in moderation.

Vitamins and Minerals

In addition to macronutrients like carbohydrates, protein, and fats, vitamins and minerals also play essential roles in blood sugar management. For example, magnesium is involved in glucose metabolism and insulin action, while chromium helps enhance insulin sensitivity. Vitamin D has also been shown to play a role in insulin secretion and glucose tolerance.

Including a variety of nutrient-dense foods in your diet ensures that you obtain adequate vitamins and minerals to support overall health and blood sugar management.

Hydration

Water is often overlooked as an essential nutrient for blood sugar management, but staying hydrated is crucial for overall health and well-being. Dehydration can lead to increased blood sugar levels and impaired insulin sensitivity, so it's essential to drink an adequate amount of water throughout the day.

Chapter 3: Feature

10 Diabetes-Friendly Snack Recipes

Snacking plays a crucial role in managing blood sugar levels for individuals with diabetes. Choosing the right snacks can help prevent blood sugar spikes and crashes while providing essential nutrients to support overall health.

In this chapter, we will explore 10 delicious and diabetes-friendly snack recipes designed to keep blood sugar stable between meals.

1. Greek Yoghurts Parfait

Ingredients:
- 1/2 cup plain Greek yoghurt
- 1/4 cup berries (such as strawberries, blueberries, or raspberries)
- 1 tablespoon chopped nuts (such as almonds or walnuts)
- 1 teaspoon honey or stevia (optional)

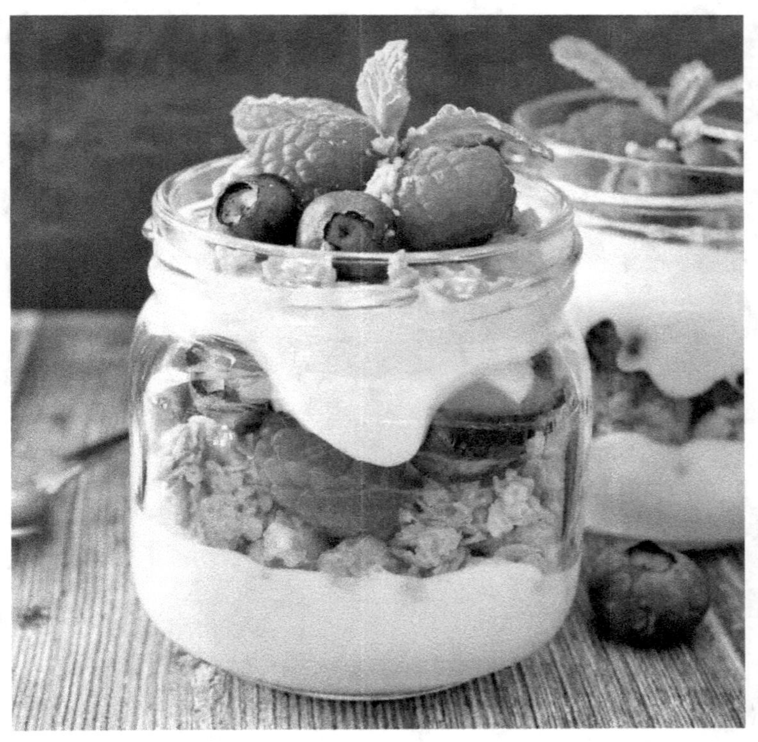

Instructions:

1. In a bowl or glass, layer Greek yoghurt, berries, and chopped nuts.

2. Drizzle with honey or sprinkle with stevia, if desired.

3. Enjoy immediately or refrigerate for later.

This Greek yoghurt parfait is packed with protein, fibre, and antioxidants, making it a satisfying and nutritious snack option for individuals managing diabetes.

2. Veggie Sticks with Hummus

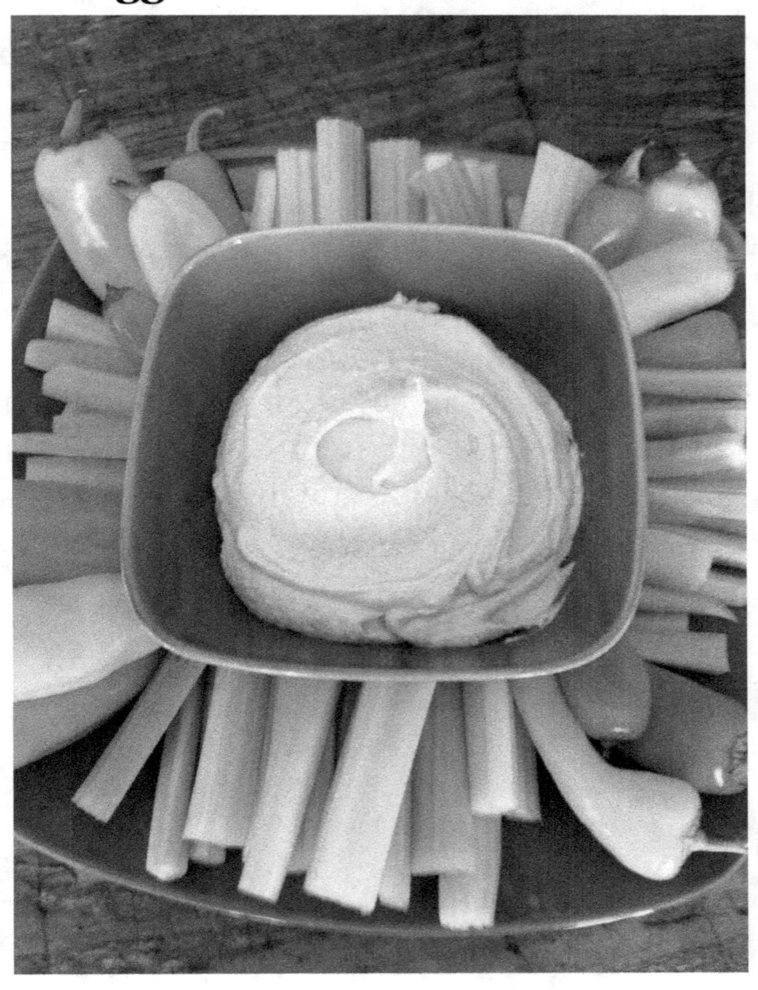

Ingredients:

- Assorted vegetable sticks (such as carrots, cucumbers, bell peppers, and celery)
- 1/4 cup hummus

Instructions:

1. Wash and cut assorted vegetables into sticks.
2. Serve with hummus for dipping.
3. Enjoy as a crunchy and flavorful snack that provides fibre, vitamins, and minerals to support blood sugar stability.

3. Avocado Toast

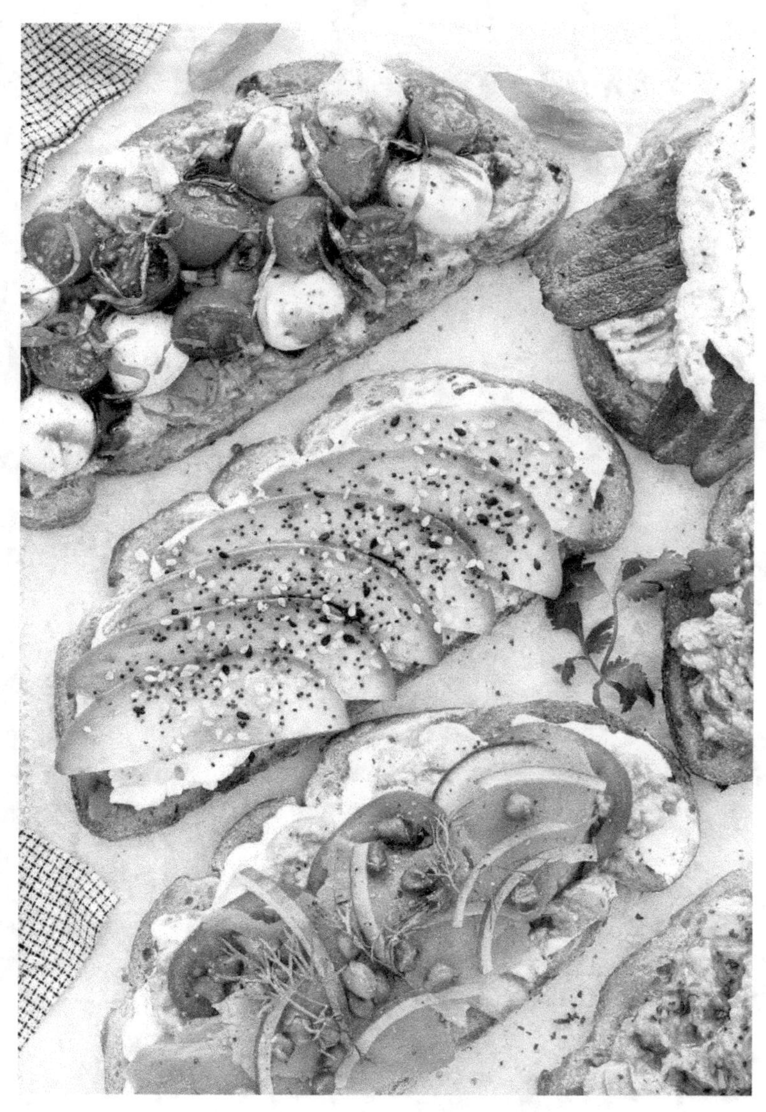

Ingredients:
- 1 slice whole-grain bread
- 1/2 ripe avocado
- Salt and pepper to taste
- Optional toppings: sliced tomatoes, sprouts, or a sprinkle of feta cheese

Instructions:
1. Toast the whole-grain bread until golden brown.
2. Mash the ripe avocado and spread it onto the toast.
3. Season with salt and pepper, and add your choice of toppings.
4. Enjoy as a satisfying and nutrient-rich snack that provides healthy fats, fibre, and vitamins.

4. Cottage Cheese and Berries

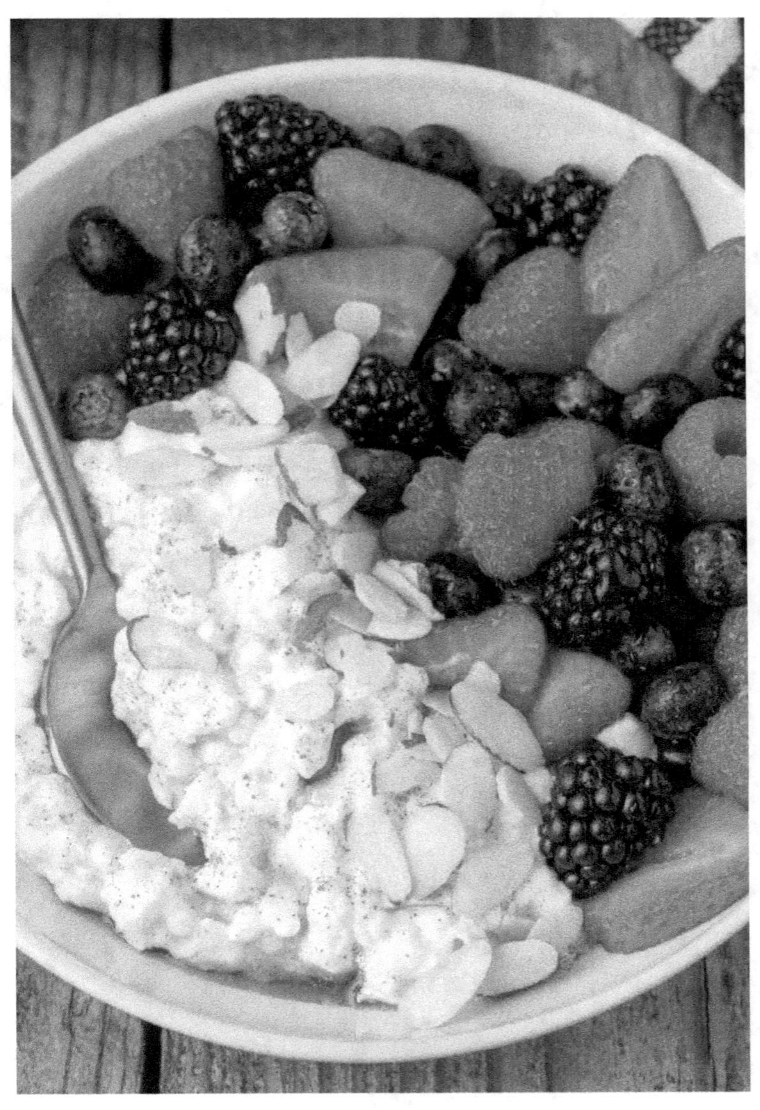

Ingredients:

- 1/2 cup cottage cheese
- 1/4 cup berries (such as strawberries, blueberries, or raspberries)
- Optional: drizzle of honey or sprinkle of stevia

Instructions:

1. Spoon cottage cheese into a bowl.

2. Top with fresh berries and drizzle with honey or sprinkle with stevia, if desired.

3. Enjoy as a protein-rich snack that also provides antioxidants and vitamins.

5. Tuna Salad Lettuce Wraps

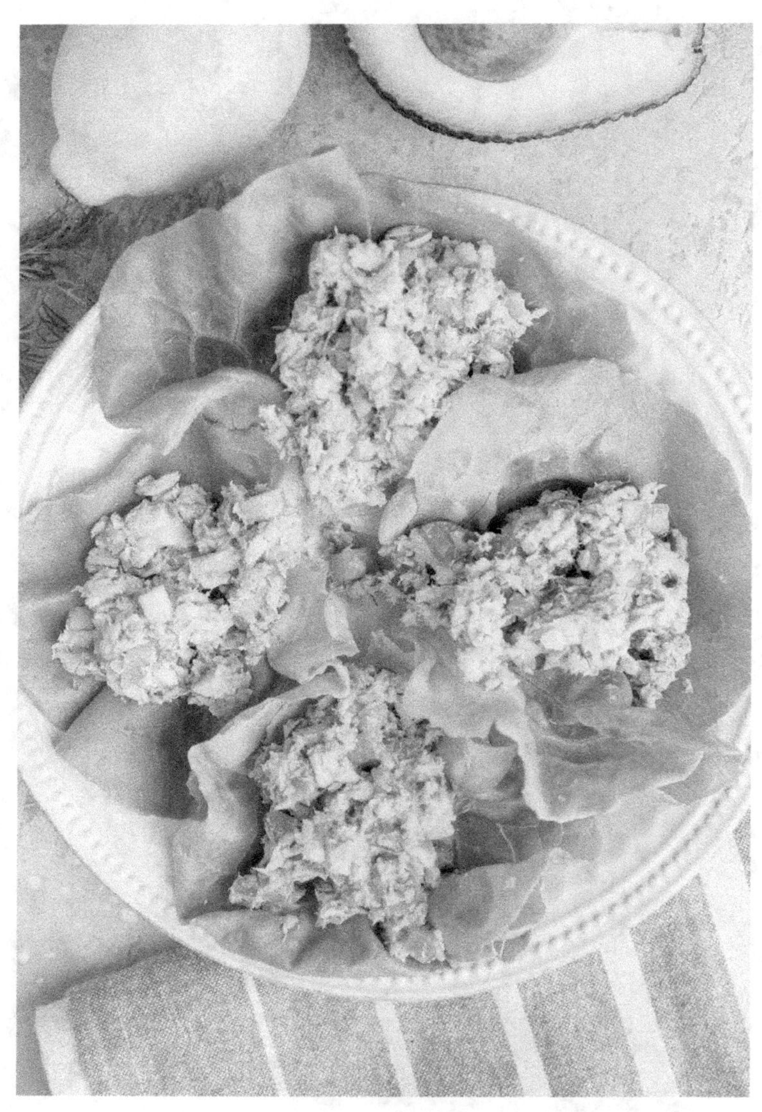

Ingredients:
- 1 can (5 ounces) tuna, drained
- 2 tablespoons plain Greek yoghurt
- 1 tablespoon chopped celery
- 1 tablespoon chopped red onion
- Salt and pepper to taste
- Lettuce leaves for wrapping

Instructions:
1. In a bowl, mix together tuna, Greek yoghurt, celery, red onion, salt, and pepper.
2. Spoon the tuna salad onto lettuce leaves and wrap to form lettuce wraps.
3. Enjoy as a protein-packed snack that is low in carbohydrates and high in essential nutrients.

6. Apple Slices with Almond Butter

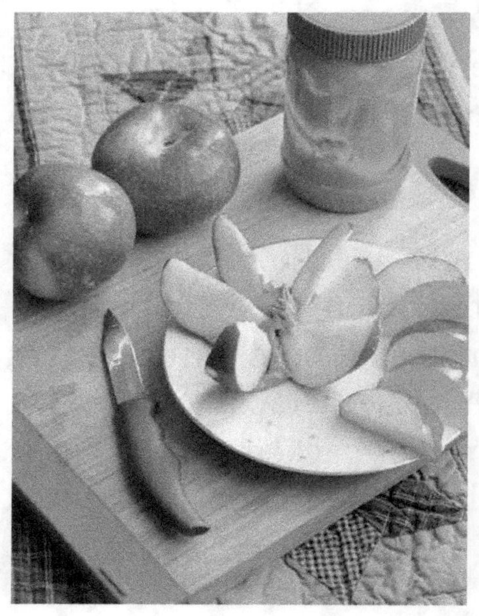

Ingredients:

- 1 medium apple, sliced
- 2 tablespoons almond butter

Instructions:

1. Wash and slice the apple into thin slices.

2. Spread almond butter onto apple slices.
3. Enjoy as a satisfying snack that provides a balance of carbohydrates, healthy fats, and fiber to support blood sugar stability.

7. Chickpea Salad

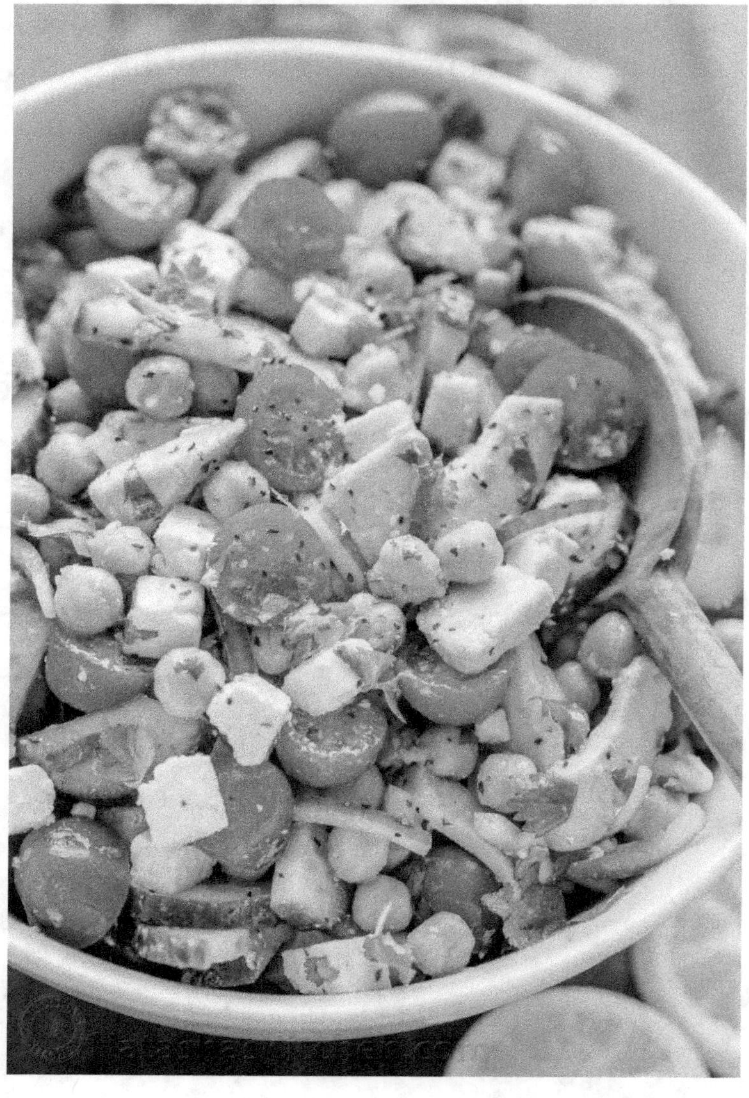

Ingredients:

- 1 can (15 ounces) chickpeas, drained and rinsed
- 1/4 cup diced cucumber
- 1/4 cup diced bell pepper
- 2 tablespoons chopped red onion
- 2 tablespoons chopped fresh parsley
- 1 tablespoon olive oil
- 1 tablespoon lemon juice
- Salt and pepper to taste

Instructions:

1. In a bowl, combine chickpeas, cucumber, bell pepper, red onion, and parsley.
2. Drizzle with olive oil and lemon juice, and season with salt and pepper.
3. Toss to combine and refrigerate for at least 30 minutes to allow flavours to meld.
4. Enjoy as a refreshing and protein-rich snack that provides fibre, vitamins, and minerals.

8. Hard-Boiled Eggs

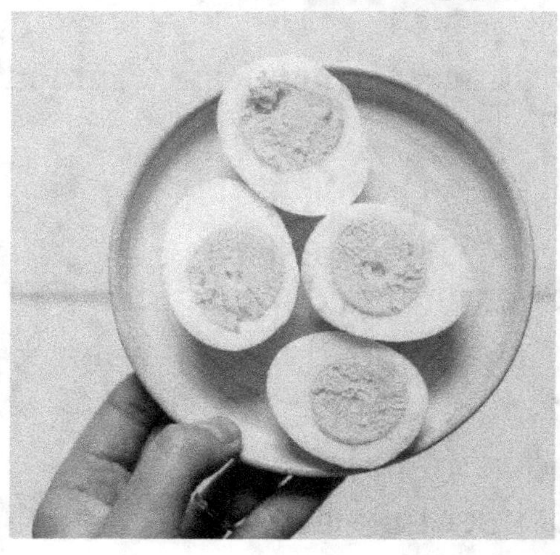

Ingredients:
- 2 eggs

Instructions:
1. Place eggs in a saucepan and cover with water.
2. Bring water to a boil, then reduce heat and simmer for 10 minutes.
3. Remove eggs from water and let cool before peeling.

4. Enjoy as a convenient and protein-rich snack that provides essential nutrients to support blood sugar stability.

9. Trail Mix

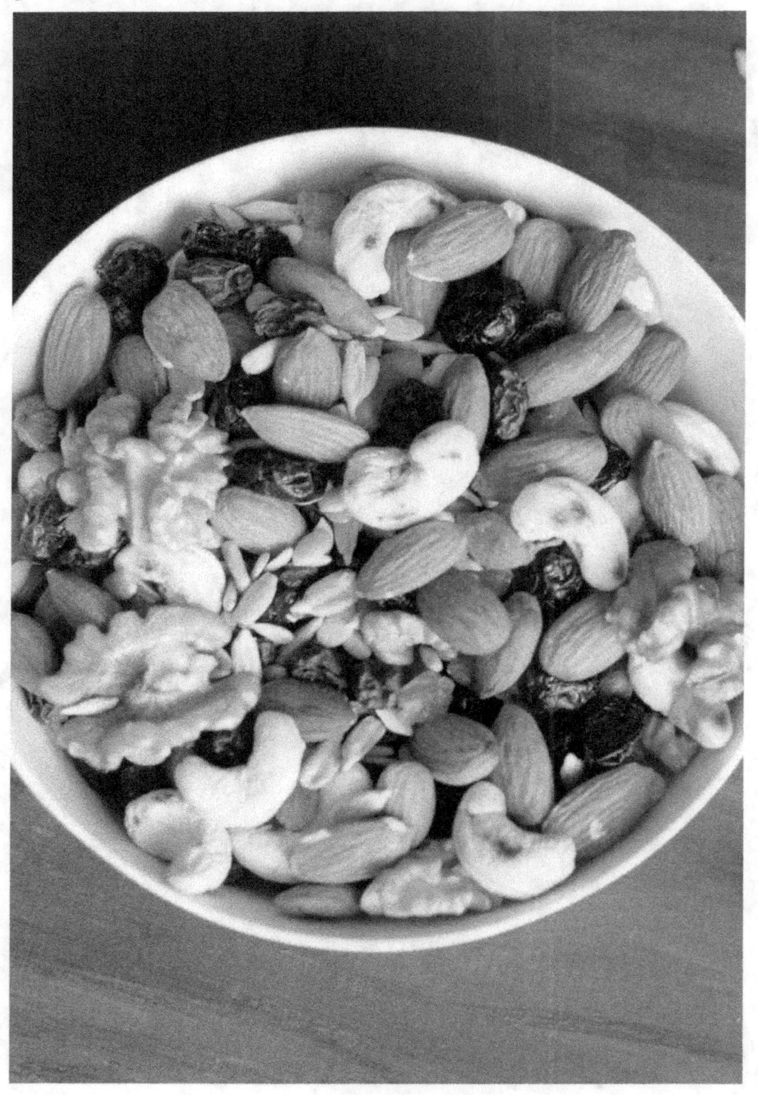

Ingredients:
- 1/4 cup mixed nuts (such as almonds, walnuts, and cashews)
- 2 tablespoons dried fruit (such as raisins, cranberries, or apricots)
- 1 tablespoon dark chocolate chips or cacao nibs

Instructions:
1. Combine mixed nuts, dried fruit, and dark chocolate chips or cacao nibs in a bowl.
2. Mix well and portion into individual servings.
3. Enjoy as a portable and nutrient-rich snack that provides a balance of carbohydrates, healthy fats, and antioxidants.

10. Rice Cake with Peanut Butter and Banana

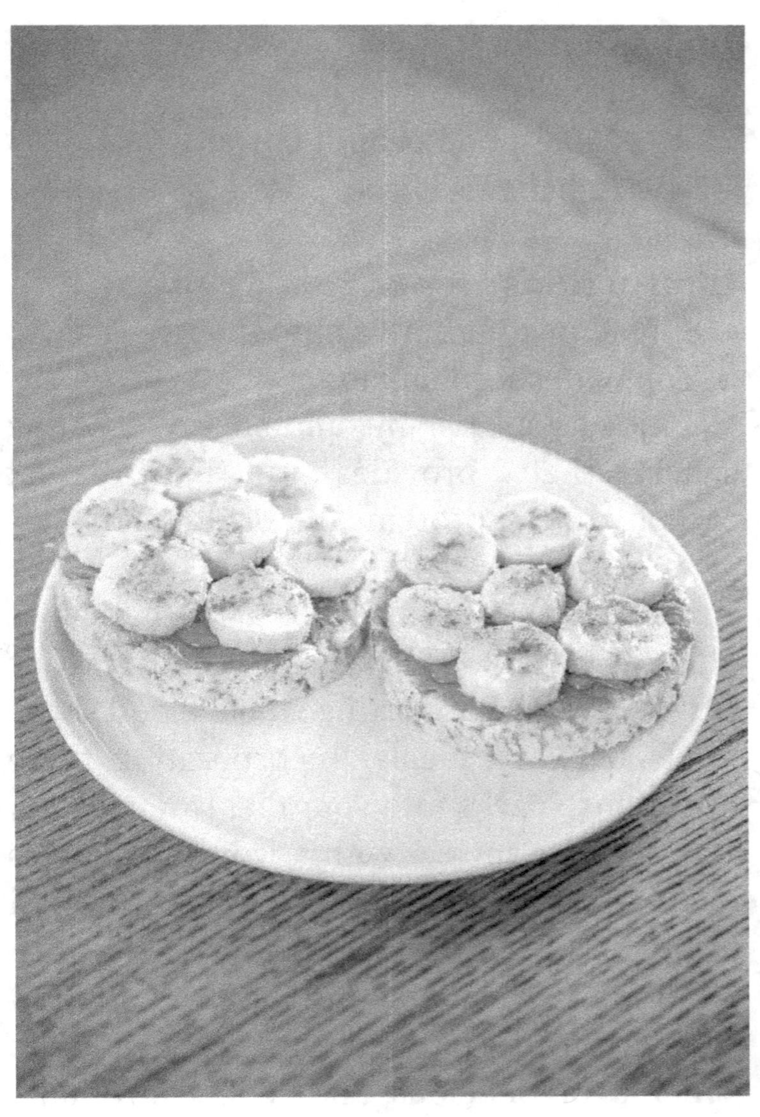

Ingredients:
- 1 rice cake
- 1 tablespoon peanut butter
- 1/2 banana, sliced

Instructions:
1. Spread peanut butter onto the rice cake.
2. Top with sliced banana.
3. Enjoy as a satisfying and energy-boosting snack that provides a balance of carbohydrates, protein, and healthy fats.

These 10 diabetes-friendly snack recipes offer a variety of options to satisfy your cravings while supporting stable blood sugar levels between meals. Incorporating these nutritious snacks into your diet can help you stay on track with your diabetes management goals and improve your overall health and well-being. Experiment with different ingredients and flavours to find your favourite combinations, and enjoy the benefits of delicious and diabetes-friendly snacking!

Chapter 4: Why These Snacks Work for Blood Sugar Stability

Balanced Macronutrients

One of the key reasons why these snacks work for blood sugar stability is their balance of macronutrients. Each snack recipe incorporates a combination of carbohydrates, protein, and healthy fats, which helps slow down the absorption of glucose into the bloodstream and prevents rapid spikes in blood sugar levels.

For example, the Greek yoghurt parfait combines protein-rich Greek yoghurt with fibre-rich berries and healthy fats from chopped nuts, creating a satisfying and balanced snack that supports blood sugar stability.

Fibre-Rich Ingredients

Fibre plays a crucial role in blood sugar management by slowing down the digestion and absorption of carbohydrates, which helps prevent rapid fluctuations in blood sugar levels. Many of the snack recipes featured in Chapter 3 include fibre-rich ingredients such as fruits, vegetables, nuts, seeds, and whole grains.

For instance, the veggie sticks with hummus provide a satisfying crunch while delivering a hefty dose of fibre from the assorted vegetable sticks and protein-rich hummus. This combination helps promote satiety and supports blood sugar stability between meals.

Low Glycemic Index

The glycemic index (GI) is a measure of how quickly a carbohydrate-containing food raises blood sugar levels. Foods with a low GI are digested and absorbed more slowly, resulting in a gradual and steady increase in blood sugar levels. Many of the snack recipes in this chapter feature ingredients with a low GI, making them ideal choices for individuals managing diabetes.

For example, the apple slices with almond butter combine the natural sweetness of apples with the healthy fats and protein from almond butter, resulting in a snack with a low GI that provides sustained energy and blood sugar stability.

Nutrient Density

Another reason why these snacks work for blood sugar stability is their nutrient density. Nutrient-dense foods provide essential vitamins, minerals, antioxidants, and phytonutrients that support overall health and well-being. By choosing snacks that are rich in nutrients, individuals can satisfy their hunger while nourishing their bodies with the building blocks of good health.

For instance, the chickpea salad features nutrient-rich ingredients such as chickpeas, cucumbers, bell peppers, and parsley, providing a powerhouse of vitamins, minerals, and antioxidants that support blood sugar stability and overall health.

Portion Control

Portion control is an essential aspect of blood sugar management for individuals with diabetes. Many of the snack recipes in this chapter are portion-controlled and designed to provide a balance of nutrients without overloading on carbohydrates or calories.

For example, the trail mix recipe combines mixed nuts, dried fruit, and dark chocolate chips in a portion-controlled serving size, allowing individuals to enjoy a satisfying and nutrient-rich snack without exceeding their carbohydrate intake goals.

Easy to Prepare

Convenience is key when it comes to maintaining healthy eating habits, especially for individuals managing diabetes. Many of the snack recipes featured in this chapter are quick and easy to prepare, making them perfect for busy lifestyles.

For instance, the hard-boiled eggs recipe requires minimal preparation and can be made ahead of time for a convenient grab-and-go snack option. Similarly, the avocado toast recipe comes together in minutes and provides a satisfying and nutrient-rich snack that can be enjoyed anytime.

These snack recipes are not only delicious but also effective tools for promoting blood sugar stability and supporting overall health for individuals managing diabetes. By incorporating a variety of nutrient-dense ingredients, balancing macronutrients, and focusing on low GI foods, these snacks provide sustained energy and help prevent rapid fluctuations in blood sugar levels.

Whether you're enjoying a Greek yoghurt parfait for breakfast, snacking on veggie sticks with hummus in the afternoon, or indulging in a rice cake with peanut butter and banana for dessert, these snacks offer a delicious and diabetes-friendly way to stay on track with your blood sugar management goals.

Experiment with different recipes and flavours to find your favourites, and enjoy the benefits of stable blood sugar levels and improved overall health. With the right snacks, managing diabetes can be both enjoyable and empowering, allowing you to live your best life with confidence and vitality.

Chapter 5: Benefits of Incorporating These Snacks into Your Diet

Blood Sugar Management

One of the primary benefits of incorporating these snacks into your diet is improved blood sugar management. By choosing snacks that are rich in fibre, protein, and healthy fats, you can help prevent rapid fluctuations in blood sugar levels and promote greater stability throughout the day. This can lead to better glycemic control and reduced risk of complications associated with poorly managed diabetes.

Sustained Energy Levels

Many of the snack recipes featured in Chapter 3 are designed to provide sustained energy levels without causing spikes or crashes in blood sugar. By opting for snacks that contain a balance of carbohydrates, protein, and healthy fats, you can fuel your body with the nutrients it needs to maintain energy levels throughout the day. This can help prevent fatigue and improve overall productivity and well-being.

Improved Safety

Snacking plays an essential role in controlling hunger and preventing overeating at meal times. The snacks featured in this chapter are not only nutritious but also satisfying, thanks to their combination of fibre, protein, and healthy fats. By incorporating these snacks into your diet, you can stay fuller for longer and reduce the likelihood of unhealthy snacking or overeating later in the day.

Nutrient Density

Another significant benefit of these snacks is their nutrient density. Many of the ingredients used in the recipes are rich in essential vitamins, minerals, antioxidants, and phytonutrients that support overall health and well-being. By choosing snacks that are nutrient-dense, you can nourish your body with the building blocks of good health and support optimal functioning of various bodily systems.

Weight Management

Maintaining a healthy weight is essential for individuals managing diabetes, as excess body weight can exacerbate insulin resistance and increase the risk of complications. The snacks featured in this chapter are designed to be portion-controlled and balanced in nutrients, making them a valuable tool for supporting weight management goals. By incorporating these snacks into your diet, you can enjoy delicious and satisfying options while supporting your efforts to achieve and maintain a healthy weight.

Convenience

In today's fast-paced world, convenience is key when it comes to maintaining healthy eating habits. Many of the snack recipes featured in this chapter are quick and easy to prepare, making them perfect for busy lifestyles. Whether you're looking for a grab-and-go option or a simple snack to enjoy at home, these recipes offer convenient solutions that fit seamlessly into your daily routine.

Variety

One of the benefits of incorporating these snacks into your diet is the opportunity to enjoy a wide variety of flavours and ingredients. From savoury options like tuna salad lettuce wraps to sweet treats like Greek yoghurt parfaits, there's something for everyone in this collection of snack recipes. By incorporating a variety of snacks into your diet, you can satisfy your cravings while still supporting your blood sugar management goals.

Improved Mood and Well-Being

Eating a balanced diet that includes a variety of nutrient-dense foods is essential for supporting mood and overall well-being. The snacks featured in this chapter are not only delicious but also packed with essential nutrients that support brain health and mood regulation. By nourishing your body with these snacks, you can support a positive mood and greater overall well-being.

Enhanced Digestive Health

Many of the snack recipes featured in this chapter are rich in fibre, which plays a crucial role in supporting digestive health. Fibre helps promote regularity, prevent constipation, and support a healthy gut microbiome. By incorporating fibre-rich snacks into your diet, you can support optimal digestive health and improve overall gastrointestinal function.

Empowerment

Perhaps one of the most significant benefits of incorporating these snacks into your diet is the sense of empowerment that comes from taking control of your health. By making conscious choices to nourish your body with nutritious snacks, you can empower yourself to better manage your diabetes and improve your overall quality of life. With the right tools and knowledge, managing diabetes can become a positive and empowering journey towards better health and well-being.

Conclusion: Empowerment Through Nutritious Snacking

In this book, we have explored the importance of blood sugar management for individuals with diabetes and the role that nutritious snacking plays in achieving this goal. From understanding the basics of diabetes and blood sugar regulation to exploring the benefits of incorporating diabetes-friendly snacks into your diet, we have covered a wide range of topics aimed at empowering you to take control of your health and well-being.

Knowledge is power, and understanding how diabetes affects the body and the importance of blood sugar management is the first step towards empowerment. By learning about the factors that influence blood sugar levels and the role that nutrition plays in managing diabetes, you can make informed decisions about your health and take proactive steps towards better blood sugar control.

One of the key messages of this book is the importance of making healthy food choices, especially when it comes to snacking. By choosing snacks that are rich in essential nutrients like fibre, protein, and healthy fats, you can support blood sugar stability and overall health. The snack recipes featured in this book are designed to provide a balance of nutrients while satisfying your cravings and keeping you feeling full and satisfied between meals.

Managing diabetes can feel overwhelming at times, but by incorporating nutritious snacks into your diet, you can take control of your health and well-being. By making conscious choices to nourish your body with foods that support blood sugar stability, you can empower yourself to better manage your diabetes and reduce the risk of complications.

Diabetes is not just about restriction and deprivation; it's also about finding joy and satisfaction in the foods you eat. The snack recipes featured in this book are not only nutritious but also delicious, offering a wide variety of flavours and ingredients to suit every taste preference. By enjoying delicious and satisfying snacks that support blood sugar stability, you can embrace the journey towards better health and well-being with positivity and enthusiasm.

Incorporating nutritious snacking into your daily routine is not just a short-term solution; it's about creating a sustainable lifestyle that supports long-term health and well-being. By making healthy eating habits a part of your everyday life, you can set yourself up for success and ensure that you continue to thrive in the years to come.

Finally, empowerment through nutritious snacking is about more than just taking care of yourself; it's also about connecting with others who share similar goals and experiences. Whether it's sharing snack ideas with friends and family or connecting with online communities and support groups, finding a sense of community can provide encouragement, motivation, and inspiration on your journey towards better health.

In conclusion, empowerment through nutritious snacking is about taking control of your health and well-being, making healthy choices that support blood sugar stability, and embracing the journey towards better health with positivity and enthusiasm. By incorporating nutritious snacks into your diet, you can empower yourself to better manage your diabetes, improve your overall quality of life, and enjoy a fulfilling and satisfying lifestyle. Remember, you have the power to take control of your health and well-being, one snack at a time. Embrace the journey, enjoy the delicious snacks, and empower yourself to live your best life with diabetes.